Stop The Shots!

Stop The Shots!

Are Vaccinations Killing Our Pets?

John Clifton

Stop The Shots! : Are Vaccinations Killing Our Pets?

Publication date: January, 2007.   ISBN: 0-9760846-2-7
Library of Congress Control Number: 2006937217

Additional copies and information:
Visit our web site at *www.StopTheShots.com* for further information, continuously updated resources on animal vaccinations, and to order additional copies of this book. Also, you will find at the very end of this book a mail-in order form for purchasing more copies.

ATTENTION VETERINARIANS, BREEDERS, CORPORATIONS, UNIVERSITIES, COLLEGES, AND PROFESSIONAL AND CHARITABLE ORGANIZATIONS: Quantity discounts are available on bulk purchases of this book for educational and gift purposes, or as premiums in fundraising efforts. Inquiries should be addressed to:

Foley Square Books
P.O. Box 20548, Park West Station
New York, NY 10025
    VOICE: 212-724-1578   FAX: 775-514-1760
    EMAIL: *info@FoleySquareBooks.com*

Contents

Acknowledgments

No man is an island – and neither are writers of books. First of all, I'd like to thank the scientists, immunologists, veterinary research organizations and the creators of and participants in the many, many studies and surveys upon which this book is based. I'm just reporting what the facts are, as currently perceived by animal experts of every stripe. Their work was far more difficult than writing this little volume, and my gratitude for their efforts knows no bounds.

It was the readers of our e-newsletter *Fighting Back: Canine Cancer Monthly* who first made me aware of the issues associated with pet vaccinations that led to the idea for a book on the subject. I thank them for writing those emails suggesting that vaccinations might have a role in pets getting cancer. It was they who put the question into my awareness: how can vaccines trigger disease?

Josée Clerens (my wife and my co-author of *Sparky Fights Back: A Little Dog's Big Battle Against Cancer*) helped me in so many ways it's daunting to try to enumerate them. Editor, research assistant, proofreader, counselor — she was all these and more. Without her there simply would be no book.

Our dog Sparky's veterinarian, Bonnie Brown, VMD, of the Ansonia Veterinary Center in New York always seemed to make room in her busy schedule to talk about pet vaccinations with me, and I thank her for her interest and encouragement.

Beatrice Ehrsam, DVM, ("Dr. Bea") was especially helpful in checking the manuscript cover to cover for any factual errors. For her taking time out from her busy practice in Chestnut Ridge, NY to consult with me about the book I am deeply grateful.

I'd also like to thank the many other veterinary professionals who were good enough to do a sanity check on the manuscript and offer corrections where there might be medical mistakes or ambiguities.

— J. C.

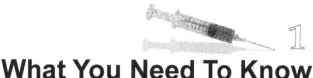

What You Need To Know

"Killing our pets?? But I thought vaccinations were to protect our animals and keep serious diseases from possibly taking their lives. I don't get it."

We all think of vaccinations as being disease *fighters*. And they are. You give your cat a distemper shot and that cat *most likely* won't get distemper. But I want to show you in this book how many believe that vaccinations can also be disease *inviters*, triggering the appearance of all sorts of maladies, from allergies to cancer.

Many owners of dogs and cats, if not most, simply aren't aware of the possible dangers inherent in immunizations. Those "annual booster shots" that seem so taken for granted have got to be questioned, in light of what is now known. The laws of localities that mandate too frequent, sometimes *annual* rabies shots have got to be abolished. We're simply giving *too many* shots *too often* for *too many* diseases (quite a few of which your pet has practically *zero* chance of getting).

If you care about your dog or your cat, you simply can't ignore the multitude of threats that vaccines could possibly pose to each and every one of them. You can't wait until it's too late. You can't say "I'll cross that bridge when I come to it." More vaccines are being injected into our pets today than ever before in our history. While it's true that rabies and some other diseases have been virtually eliminated in our pet population, our animals are coming down with more allergies than ever before, more stress, and most notably: more *cancer* than they were getting even a few years ago! One recent study shows that in the state of New York the cancer rate among dogs has increased 150% in the last four years. This, while our air and water are actually improving.

Why?

If you don't know the specific dangers being claimed, it's time you educated yourself. That's what this book is about. I'll explain what vaccines are and how they work. I'll show you what leading immunology experts are recommending – that you can cut down on the frequency of shots and still protect your pet. I will show you how to determine what inoculations are completely unnecessary for your particular dog or cat. I'll explain how, according to much current thinking, vaccines lower the immune system, leaving your pet vulnerable to serious – sometimes fatal – diseases. I'll give you the facts. I'll relate the findings of leading veterinarians, experts, and the results of pertinent surveys. I'll tell you why many breeders have abandoned vaccinations completely.

I'm not going to tell you to never again vaccinate your pet (although a good many are choosing that route nowadays). On the other hand, I'm not going to tell you, as many believe, that vaccinations are the best way to go. But I hope to lay out the pros and cons so that you can make up your own mind as to what path you will follow.

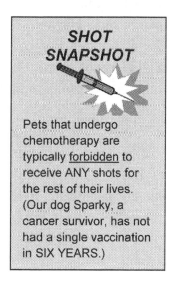

SHOT SNAPSHOT

Pets that undergo chemotherapy are typically forbidden to receive ANY shots for the rest of their lives. (Our dog Sparky, a cancer survivor, has not had a single vaccination in SIX YEARS.)

It's my intention that after reading this book you'll be able to make more informed, intelligent decisions about which vaccinations to give, which to avoid, and why. I'm going to try to keep it simple and direct; if you're looking for a highly detailed exhaustive study on the subject, this is not that book.

I *don't* want to turn you against your veterinarian! But I *do* intend to turn you into a "better educated consumer" as far as vaccinations are concerned. No medical professional is infallible. That's why second opinions were invented. Some veterinarians, I admit, seem to be totally unconcerned about possible dangers, sending out those "Time For Max's Annual Booster Shots" notices with the regularity of dentists who mail "Regular Checkup Time" postcards. Other vets (not always as visible) are as concerned as I about the permanent damage that vaccinations could be capable of causing. I consider the fact that I am not myself a veterinarian an advantage in writing this book, since I have no colleagues to defend and no professional axe to grind.

So I'm going to make some suggestions about how you can put the brakes on those vets who are inclined to overdo the shots – without seeming to challenge their competence. Remember that a veterinarian can be a perfectly ethical individual, but is not financially motivated to discontinue – or give fewer – inoculations. It's currently estimated that giving shots constitutes

50% of a typical veterinarian's practice. Some have even suggested that veterinarians over-vaccinate because they profit from treating the diseases caused by their over-vaccinating!

Well, all of this has created quite a controversy. And here's the punch – if veterinarians disagree on the benefits and dangers of vaccines, how is a poor dog or cat owner going to figure it all out? A lot will be up to *you*. If you feel your doc needs to be reined in, *you* will have to take the reins!

As editor of a monthly "e-zine" on canine cancer, and co-author of a book dealing with that subject, I get heart-wrenching letters nearly every day from dog owners devastated by the recent diagnosis of cancer in their beloved best friends. And I'm sure that owners of cancer-cats are just as devastated. Often, the disease is described as incurable.

I have been there myself. I know that empty, helpless feeling. If this book can prevent even one of these cases, it will have been worth the effort. But I hope these words help to sound an alert to all pet owners everywhere: "Learn the facts! Beware the dangers! And – until you've sorted it all out for yourself and come to your own conclusion – *stop the shots!*"

So, let's take a closer look at vaccines...

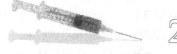

How Vaccines Work

"What's to know? You get a shot for a certain disease and it protects you against that disease."

Well, that seems true. But, without getting technical, let's go into it a little bit more. To understand the possible *dangers* of vaccines, which are what this book is about, it will help you to know just what vaccines are.

The word "vaccine" is derived from *vacca*, Latin for "cow." That's because the first vaccine (developed by Edward Jenner in England in 1796) came from cowpox, a disease in cows, the virus of which was developed into human small-pox vaccine. Today the term is used for any preparation administered by mouth, injection, or nasal spray that is designed to produce *antibodies* against any one of a number of diseases.

Vaccines are typically made using the viruses or bacteria of a particular disease. Sometimes these microorganisms have been killed, other times they've only been weakened a bit (more about this later).

For example, a human flu shot will contain flu virus (typically a "killed" virus). The idea is to introduce a small quantity of the disease into the body. This, in turn, stimulates the immune system to respond, be the virus dead carcasses or live little organisms. Little guys called "antigens" go running around sounding the alarm that a stranger has entered the body. They inform other little guys that turn into little warriors called "antibodies." These antibodies are specifically trained on the spot to fight the specific virus.

But, after they've destroyed the invader, the antibodies don't fold up their tents. They hang around – just in case more of those enemies come back. Basically that's what immunity is – having those antibodies around, ready to nip that virus in the bud should it ever return.

Additionally, the immune system puts a profile of each individual enemy it encounters into its own *enemy database,* called "memory cells." These cells can survive for years, even after the antibody warriors have died natural deaths, thus prolonging immunity.

When a person or an animal gets a vaccination, it starts with what I think of as a little war in the body. The immune system gets real *busy*. Getting busy takes energy. All those antigens responding to the alarm! All those antibodies being created! Many contend that this consumption of energy and resources creates a temporary *weakness*. We say the immune system has been *lowered*. Or, worse, *compromised*. So that's the paradox: in order to "strengthen" immunity, the system has to be weakened for a time. Almost all agree on this. It can be clearly demonstrated that the number of white cells in the blood is diminished after a vaccination.

And many knowledgeable folks contend that during that "window

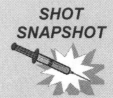

SHOT SNAPSHOT

There are <u>three</u> basic types of immunity–

<u>Mucosal</u> immunity works in the mucous linings of the digestive, urinary, respiratory and mammary tracts preventing invaders from entering the body.

<u>Humoral</u> immunity works in the body's fluid sources – mainly the blood – producing antibodies against invaders.

<u>Cellular</u> immunity works in the individual cells, keeping records from past experiences with invaders, and recognizing them if they should ever return. It is this system that produces the <u>symptoms</u> of disease (fever, diarrhea, rashes, etc.)

of weakness," bad things can happen! It's hard for an army to fight on too many fronts at once – resources are stretched to the breaking point. And so it is with the immune system. Remember, it doesn't know that this is just a vaccine it's dealing with; it thinks it's the real disease – and responds accordingly. And if this army called the immune system has to deal with *multiple* enemies, well, you get the idea.

Other enemies that were kept in check before can now get a toehold. That's why you should know about recommendations for spacing out vaccinations. Veterinary immunologists have already constructed carefully worked out regimens called "protocols," which specify what vaccines to give and at what age, and at what intervals to repeat each specific shot. I'll get to that later.

A veterinarian recently told me about seeing a puppy, "Alfie," who had previously been vaccinated by another vet. According to the dog's medical record, the first vet had given the poor little thing *three shots at once* when he was only a few weeks old. That's creating a pretty major war, and at a time when the animal's immune system wasn't fully developed. I predict that Alfie will probably get cancer or another serious disease sooner or later. I hope I'm wrong, but I'm not optimistic. Believe it or not, there exists a *"seven-in-one"* vaccine cocktail, and it's not un-usual to hear that this concoction is given to very young puppies!

Some say, *"So?* What's wrong with that? It's been shown that the immune system is per-fectly capable of fending off many diseases at once."

Others say, "Are you kidding? The effects of over-vaccinating might not appear at *first*. In fact, they may not be felt for several *generations* – but the damage is done now."

Enough controversy? Want more? Besides the actual viral or bacterial organisms in vac-cines, there can be other stuff in there as well. Many vaccines contain "adjuvants." Adjuvants are immune system boosters, put there to encourage the body to fight the disease the vac-cine is meant to prevent. Adjuvants "stimulate" (irritate!) the immune system, basically saying "Hey guys! This is a bad thing that's happening here! You better get busy and start protecting yourself!" Sometimes the adjuvant can cause inflammation at the site of the injection. The inflammation causes free radicals (dangerously incomplete atoms) to circulate in the area, which can mess up the DNA in the inflamed region, and even cause cancer at the place where the needle went in. Such a sarcoma ("site-specific") is often deadly.

Cats are particularly susceptible to "Vaccine Associated Sarcomas" ("VAS") – cancers that appear at the site of the injection. Many veterinarians instead of giving cats their vaccinations between the shoulder blades, give them in their rear legs instead (see page 76). This is done because the legs can be readily amputated if cancer develops. Neat, huh?

Preservatives can also be added to vaccines. In the past, mercury was often used for this purpose, producing the results you might expect from such a toxic substance, and creating a great public outcry. Mercury use, I'm informed, is not as prevalent today (although I've just read reports of a *recent* human flu vaccine containing mercury being approved by the FDA). But – what might be the *next* additive that is discovered to be in there and found to be dangerous? You see why I keep on insisting you consider giving a *minimum* of shots?

Young mammals automatically carry immunities, transferred to them by their mothers' milk. Nature has provided that immunity to tide them over until their immune systems mature. One of the tricky things is that we can't be sure exactly how long the natural protection is lasting. When it fades, a puppy or kitten will be susceptible to all kinds of diseases, many of them extremely dangerous.

Vaccinations against Parvo, distemper, and other diseases are usually deemed necessary during this period, and it gets to be a crucial matter as to just what to give and when.

Be careful! That's my message. Many believe that the fate of the dog or cat's health later in life can be sealed by the immune measures that are taken at this early stage.

And consider this no-brainer – an animal will never get a disease it's not exposed to. A puppy that isn't living with other animals and has no contact with wild animals has practically no chance of getting rabies. Why would you vaccinate any earlier than you need to? Use your common sense.

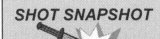

SHOT SNAPSHOT

"Most Pet Owners Don't Have a Clue"

In her popular agility classes, Marcy Pratt of Lido Beach teaches dog owners to zoom their corgis through tunnels and sail their Australian shepherds over jumps. But as she chatted with the handlers on the sidelines, she realized there was another area they needed help navigating.

"I found that most of them had their dogs vaccinated for everything, every year," Pratt says, even though the trend in veterinary medicine has been to tailor vaccine programs to a dog's lifestyle and risk. "And I had a couple of students whose dogs had had adverse reactions, including one that almost died."

– Newsday, April 3, 2006

Again, more about this later, when I'll talk about the *unnecessary* shots that are being given every day. I don't consider this topic controversial. There is certainly no benefit from a vaccine for a disease your pet stands no chance of ever getting.

But first, let's look at what diseases your pet *could* get as a result of over-vaccinating...

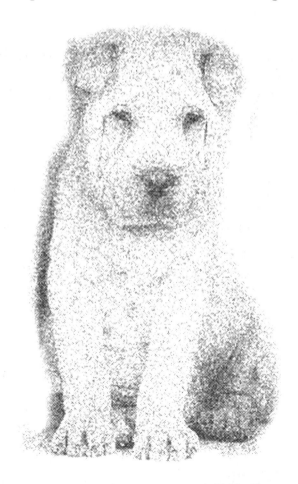

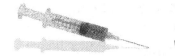

Diseases Vaccinations Can <u>Cause</u>

"I'd like to know just how likely it is that my dog or cat will get a disease from a vaccination. And what diseases might they get?"

The list of diseases that vaccinations might *possibly* cause would be large indeed, since the door to most *all* diseases is left open by immune systems that have been compromised by vaccines. Here are *just a few* of the diseases that some have suspected in actual cases to have been directly linked to vaccines:

> Cancers (various types)
> Paralysis
> Allergies (all sorts – respiratory, skin, etc.)

Leukemia
Liver damage
Lupus and various auto-
immune
disorders
Parvovirus
Hepatitis
Parainfluenza
Leptospirosis
Chronic Renal
(Kidney)
Failure

At least one study suggests that vaccines can cause or trigger diseases *directly*. There was a survey done in the UK in 1996, "The Canine Health Census." This survey was drawn up by leading veterinary immunology experts from the United States, England and Australia. The results basically demonstrated that the *vast ma-*

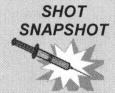

SHOT SNAPSHOT

Vaccine-Associated Feline Sarcoma–

–A cancer of the connective tissues beneath the skin that occurs at the site of an immunization. It happens in a small number of cats, but is very aggressive and difficult to control. Since the late 1980s, veterinarians have noticed inflammatory reactions in cats between three and five weeks after a vaccination. The vaccine reaction starts as a small lump at the site of the injection...

Some of the reactive cats later developed an aggressive connective tissue tumor, called sarcoma.

— from a 2001 press release, North Carolina State University *jority* of dogs that came down with various diseases came down with the disease within 90 days after a vaccination!

The way I figure it (and I'm no great mathematician), since three months is a quarter of a year, the odds would indicate that on any given day of the year there would be no more than a 25% chance of a vaccination occurring within the previous 90 days, assuming one shot-day per year. But the survey showed that of all dogs that contracted a disease 55% to 100% of them (depending on the disease) had had vaccinations within the 90 day period. The diseases included distemper, parvovirus, hepatitis and leptospirosis. By the way, leptospirosis cases *always* showed a vaccination occurring in the previous 90 day period. *Every single case* showed some sort of shot given in the past three months!

Something is going on here.

You see now why I say that vaccinations might be "disease *inviters*." Readers of our newsletter have suggested to me that in each case of cancer, you will find a vaccination in the not-so-distant past. I haven't found a study on this – however, I don't discount it as a theory. Our Sparky had received a vaccination 6 months before his diagnosis of lymphoma, and was (in my current, more informed opinion) definitely an over-vaccinated animal, especially in his puppy-hood. No more, thank heaven.

It is suspected that certain purebred dogs are particularly genetically disposed to adverse reactions. In a recent study conducted by veterinarian George Moore of Purdue University, dachshunds, pugs, Boston terriers, miniature pinschers and Chihuahuas showed higher rates of adverse events than other breeds.

So, should a pet owner stop *all* vaccinations? *Some? Any?* Which ones?

Let's explore the answers...

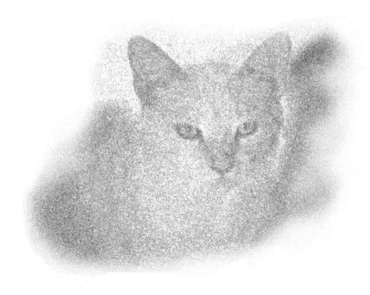

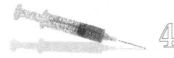

Which And Which Not?

"When in doubt about giving a particular shot, the logical thing would be to give it, right? You never know, so it's always better to play it safe, I say. More is better, right?"

Wrong.

That would almost be like taking pills for every disease there *is*, just in case you might have one of them. Be selective! In one respect vaccinations are not that different from any other medical treatment – there are always risks that come along with the benefits. An animal overwhelmed with vaccinations will likely be far worse off than one who has received *no* vaccinations, many would argue.

Some dog and cat breeders these days are saying that they no longer vaccinate puppies or kittens at all, and claim that, on balance, they're experiencing fewer rather than more health problems. Many opine that vaccinations actually *weaken* the breed, due to the fact that animals never get the opportunity to fight off certain diseases naturally. When young puppies and kittens get a disease and fight it off without the aid of vaccines, their immune systems, it is argued, are left far stronger than if they had been protected by vaccines and never got the disease. This bodes for stronger offspring, and more and more breeders, it seems, are becoming aware of this.

Despite the title of this book, I'm not personally advocating stopping *all* shots. But I can certainly see why some are going that way. A reader of our newsletter *Fighting Back: Canine Cancer Monthly* wrote me an email to say that he has dogs, cats, and horses and none of them has *ever* gotten a vaccination, nor have any of them *ever* contracted cancer. I'd venture a guess that he lives in the country, away from the dangers of city life where diseases are so readily communicable. Still, such cases are intriguing. Other readers send similar reports. I know of no studies specifically focusing on pets that have *never* received vaccinations – but would certainly welcome one.

There seems to be little doubt in the veterinary world (particularly among holistic vets) that vaccines can cause specific health problems in dogs and cats. Concerns have been raised for some time now. In their book "The Holistic Guide For A Healthy Dog" (1995), authors Wendy Volhard and Kerry Brown DVM wrote:

> *Immunologists are finding a direct correlation between the increase in autoimmune and chronic disease states and the overuse of vaccines. Breeders have had entire litters wiped out after using Parvo vaccines. Some breeds, notably Rottweillers, who were subjected to weekly doses of Parvo vaccine in the late 1980s, were riddled with bone cancers and died around the age of 4 years. The Lyme disease vaccine is thought to have been responsible for the collapse of some dogs' immune systems, and a recent study at Cornell University suggests that treating the disease is less risky than getting the vaccine.*

I receive emails from many breeders reporting similar sounding experiences. Apparently in the minds of many "shots" equals "cancer."

Michelle T. Bernard, author of "Raising Cats Naturally," is a holistic breeder who wrote a long article (for *blakkatz.com*) on the topic of cat vaccinations. I find this comment typical of many breeders:

> *Except for what's required by law (rabies) most of my cats are not vaccinated. I haven't vaccinated a cat in over ten years... I take the approach that if one of my cats gets sick, I'll deal with it.*

Many, however, particularly city dwellers, aren't willing to go that far. They would rather vaccinate, but with a careful, judicious approach.

So, barring total abstinence, what shots should you give, and which should you avoid? That depends on several factors, including your pet's environment, lifestyle, and medical history. But when considering any particular shot, the immediate question you should ask yourself is: what are the chances my pet will ever be exposed to this disease? Just remember, one size does *not* fit all!

Later in this chapter, I've created a series of yes-or-no questions for you to use as a guide. But, first, let's see just what vaccines are being produced and administered these days.

Here is a partial list of diseases you could possibly vaccinate your pet against. Vaccine manufacturers are coming up with new vaccines all the time, so this is not an all-inclusive list, but it should give you some idea of what's out there today:

Typical Vaccines

DOGS	CATS
Rabies	Rabies
Canine distemper	Panleukopenia
Parvovirus	("feline distemper,"
Bordetella	"cat typhoid," "cat
("kennel cough")	fever")
Adenovirus	Infectious peritonitis
(Hepatitis)	Rhinotracheitis
Parainfluenza	Feline Parvovirus
Coronavirus	Calcivirus
Leptospirosis	Bordetella
Lyme disease	Feline leukemia
Giardia	Dermaphytosis
	Giardia

Rabies (Latin for "rage") is a viral disease that causes acute encephalitis* in animals and people. In humans, rabies is almost always fatal once full-blown symptoms have developed, but prompt vaccination after exposure usually prevents symptoms from developing. Rabies shots for dogs and cats are usually required by law in the United States, as well as many foreign

---

* inflammation of the brain

countries. The laws are intended ultimately not to protect the animals, but to protect humans who could possibly be infected from animal bites. Human rabies is quite rare in the United States. Only 27 cases have been reported in people in the United States since 1990. 90% of rabies occurs in wild animals. In Asia, Africa and Latin America, however, rabies remains a substantial threat to animals and people. Bats commonly carry rabies.

Distemper and Parvovirus both cause severe vomiting and diarrhea, and are often fatal in young animals.

Bordetella, or "kennel cough," is contracted in kennels and shelters, and is considered curable with antibiotics.

Adenovirus and Parainfluenza are respiratory illnesses.

Coronavirus is a highly contagious disease infecting the intestinal tract.

Leptospirosis is a contagious, possibly fatal disease often affecting the liver or kidney.

Lyme disease in animals is similar to the disease in humans, and symptoms can include fever, lameness and soreness, listlessness, loss of appetite, swollen glands and joints.

Feline Parvovirus is a cause of feline panleukopenia.

Rhinotracheitis is a common upper respiratory infection similar to a cold in humans.

Calcivirus produces ulcerations in the mouth. Some strains may also produce relatively mild signs of upper respiratory tract disease.

Giardia is a microscopic parasite difficult to get rid of. A study of cats deliberately infected with the parasite done by the Colorado State University indicated that the vaccine was *totally* ineffective. It was suggested, however, that the vaccine might have a beneficial effect on cats *naturally* infected.

Hmm...

Picking Your Shots

Well! That's quite a menu! Which vaccines should you give and which not? For *starters*, you can weed the list out by answering "yes" or "no" to the following questions. That will leave you with a shorter list to evaluate further.

Yes or No – ?

Did I just adopt my dog from a shelter or just get my pet from a breeder? [If "YES," then the shelter or breeder has possibly already vaccinated for bordetella. Check to make sure.

Don't repeat this shot. In fact, check previous shot records for *all* rescues and puppies.]

Will I be boarding my pet with other dogs or cats? [If "NO," omit bordetella.]

Does my pet live in, or will she be traveling to an area where Lyme disease is endemic? [If "NO," eliminate Lyme disease.]

Do I want to keep vaccinations to the bare minimum, eliminating shots for diseases that usually can be cured – and paying special attention to my pet's general health? [DOGS: If "YES," eliminate all but rabies, parvovirus and canine distemper. CATS: If "YES," eliminate all but rabies, panleukopenia and rhinotracheitis/calcivirus.]

NOTE: Many choose to vaccinate puppies and kittens with these "core" vaccines only (according to recommended schedules) up until their pets reach 12 months old – then discontinue shots entirely thereafter for the life of the animal.

Do I want to eliminate shots that have not been proven to offer protection? [If "YES," eliminate Giardia, Canine Coronavirus, and Feline infectious peritonitis.]

Do I want to eliminate <u>all</u> shots, except what the law requires? [If "YES," eliminate all but rabies (unless you live in a place with some peculiar animal laws.) Then start concentrating on keeping your animal in top health, using diet, supplements, exercise and regular checkups (We'll get into that later).]

Okay, now the question is – do I *repeat* the shots? And how often?

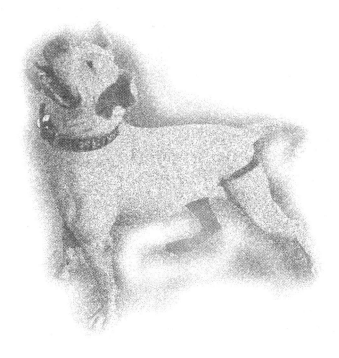

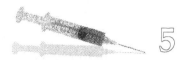

All In The Timing: How Frequent?

"Doesn't every shot sooner or later wear out? Don't I have to repeat them every year? I hear so much about 'annual booster shots'."

Please *forget* the phrase "annual booster shots!" These three words just don't belong together. Regular *annual shots* don't make any sense – and should be completely abolished. So why, then, are some veterinarians still sending out those "Time For Your Annual Shots" notices?

The American Veterinary Medical Association, in its *Principles of Vaccination* guidelines (2001) states:

> *Unnecessary stimulation of the immune system does not result in enhanced disease resistance, and may increase the risk of adverse post-vaccination events.*

In other words, if your pet is already immune to something, giving an additional shot for it won't improve matters. On the contrary.

Scheduling vaccinations is a matter of repeating shots at the *widest* sensible intervals. Never repeat a shot if it's clear that the previous one is still capable of offering protection. Personally, I would err on the side of waiting too long, rather than not waiting long enough.

Truth be told, the facts aren't in on just how long individual vaccinations remain effective. And who knows if the same time periods apply to all animals, all breeds? There are studies being done, and more is known today than, say, ten years ago. But one thing is clear – the more this topic is studied, the more we are finding that shots last *longer* that we originally thought. It's now claimed that "live virus" shots last for *life* and never have to be repeated. Distemper shots are always "live virus," so can't we assume that they never have to be repeated? Am I missing something? Most other vaccinations last several years. There is a "killed" rabies vaccine now that is labeled as lasting "three years." I wouldn't be surprised to hear one day that this has been upped to five or seven years – or life.

Studies done at the University of Wisconsin's Veterinary Teaching Hospital show that vaccines for Parvovirus, distemper, and hepatitis protect for *at least* seven years. This should tell you something about the value of "annual boosters" for at least these three diseases.

Immunologists have devised protocols that incorporate the best current data. They've come up with standardized schedules for vaccination-giving. One noted veterinarian who's been working on this for years is Jean Dodds DVM. (The fact that health risks are associated with vaccinations is nothing new – it's just that recently the facts are becoming better known.) Dr. Dodds is a minimalist. Her schedule for puppy vaccinations is bare bones (no pun intended). And that's good. And clear. She doesn't include what you might refer to as "optional" or "non core" vaccinations, such as kennel cough, Lyme disease and the like. If you think you need to immunize your pup against anything over and above distemper, parvovirus and rabies, that's an individual matter, and often could be an informed choice you make with your veterinarian – taking your pet, its area and lifestyle into consideration. Or it could be simply having your bill padded. I'll say no more than that.

Except to say that Dr. Dodds' protocol, having been largely ignored for many years, is now the standard being taught in virtually all of the veterinary colleges in the U.S. You would think it would at last have found universal use. You would think that every single veterinarian would now know enough, and care enough, to never again give gratuitous vaccinations for diseases our pets are unlikely to come into contact with. You would think that the concept of annual boosters would have been abandoned. You would think.

Here is Dr. Dodds' protocol for the vaccination of puppies. Notice how *simple* it is!

Vaccination Protocol / Jean Dodds DVM	
Age of Pups	Vaccine Type
9 - 10 weeks	Distemper + Parvovirus, MLV (e.g. Intervet Progard Puppy DPV)
14 weeks	Same as above
16 –18 weeks (optional)	Same as above
20 weeks or older, if allowable by law	Rabies
1 year	Distemper + Parvovirus, MLV
1 year	Rabies, killed 3-year product (give 3-4 weeks *apart* from distemper/parvovirus booster)

"MLV" indicates "modified live virus." Note that the rabies shot is separated from other shots by 3-4 weeks. I would also consider separating the distemper and parvo shots by at least a week. It goes against my grain to give two shots on the same visit, although I offer no hard data to back up my concern. Talk to your vet about it.

Dr. Dodds adds the following instructions for follow-ups:

> *Perform vaccine antibody titers for distemper and parvovirus annually thereafter. Vaccinate for rabies virus according to the law, except where circumstances indicate that a written waiver needs to be obtained from the primary care veterinarian. In that case, a rabies antibody titer can also be performed to accompany the waiver request.*

A "titer" test can prove to the authorities that your animal doesn't need a new vaccination (booster), that the old one is still doing the job just fine, thank you very much. The test might cost more than the shot – but isn't it worth it if you can avoid even one single unnecessary vaccination? Yes, it is. Especially a rabies shot. (For more on titers, see page 47.)

When you receive those annual postcards from your veterinarian to come on in and get those annual boosters, first determine if there will be any shots given that aren't really necessary, such as, say, bordetella – which is considered a curable disease. Then ask how it can be shown that the old shot for, say, rabies isn't still protecting.

Don't get me wrong; it's always good to get an annual *checkup*. These visits are a good way to detect trouble early. It's just that the yearly ritual doesn't have to include *shots*. So, when you get one of those little reminders, make the appointment, but question the shots.

So now – you're going to have your pet vaccinated (or revaccinated). Time to prepare...

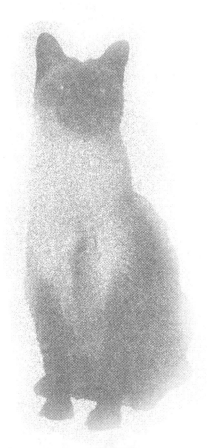

<u>Before</u> You Vaccinate

"If my animal is in good health, there's nothing special I need to do to prepare her for a shot. Or is there?"

There are things you can – and should – do to prime your pet for a shot. Mainly, actively boost the immune system. And secondly, make sure he's not under any special stress.

Most animal health professionals would agree that the single most effective thing you can do to improve and maintain your pet's health is to feed a healthy diet. Here is where some common sense and, I think, balance comes into play. There are more opinions, it seems, about what constitutes a healthy diet than there are opinions about vaccines!

You've probably heard by now that commercial pet food is bad, bad, bad! Well, again, lots of it is, but not all. The chief culprit in commercial food is "animal byproducts" – which can mean stuff coming from the bodies of dead (perhaps diseased) pets, or their ashes. Then there are preservatives and other chemicals, and lots of other questionable ingredients. Much has been written on the evils of commercial food, and I'll not go into it here – that's another book. But some careful searches can turn up pet food that's acceptable – even good. All the bad publicity seems to have had at least some effect on what's being sold.

Then you're no doubt aware of the *natural raw* diet for dogs – all uncooked meat like wolves eat in the wild, along with food-processed vegetables imitating the stomach contents of their prey. This diet has many adherents, and they swear by it, claiming especially healthy animals. Opponents say that raw meat is dangerous, containing unhealthy bacteria and parasites. And many point out that wolves in the wild aren't all that healthy anyway.

Then there are *macrobiotic* diets. I know owners who feed their dogs almost nothing but brown rice and a few certain grains and vegetables – no meat at all! It appears to me that what's going on is people mistaking dogs for either other people or wolves. We're projecting ourselves, often, onto the animals. It gets kind of crazy, I think. Dogs are dogs – domesticated animals, who if set free in the world and left to their own devices would probably eat most anything they could find or kill. And the same, or course, goes for cats.

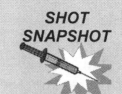

SHOT SNAPSHOT

"Vaccines clog our lymphatic system and lymph nodes with large protein molecules which have not been adequately broken down by our digestive processes. This is why vaccines are linked to allergies."
      – Dr. Joseph Mercola

Digestion prepares what you eat for the bloodstream. Anything in a hypodermic goes directly into the blood, without that benefit.

When I was a kid (in the 1940's and 50's) our family dog, a terrier mix, was fed only a cereal-type dry commercial food called "Gro-Pup," occasional leftovers from our table, and a MilkBone dog biscuit once in a while. Of course you know where I'm going with this: He lived to be 16 years old, healthy to the end. And I have no memory of his being vaccinated, though he probably had a rabies shot as a puppy.

Personally, I weigh in on the side of variety and balance. Extreme diets – *all* this or *all* that make no sense to me. We feed our dog the basic "raw diet" as a foundation, but don't follow it stringently. Depending on what we're eating, he'll get perhaps some other wholesome "people" food as well – cooked or raw.

So what's a healthy diet for your dog or cat? That depends on you, and, as I say, it's a topic not within the scope of this book. What I *would* like to touch on is the area of foods and other factors that build the immune system. If (a) you choose to vaccinate, and (b) vaccines tax the immune system, many animal health professionals suggest that you give a special buildup beginning a few weeks *before* the shot is to be given, and continue for a few weeks *afterward.* Here are some immunity-building suggestions you might consider discussing with your veterinarian:

Vitamins. Your animal might have a Vitamin B deficiency, and some vaccines might need that Vitamin B to be effective. Also, stress might lower B levels. So consider giving B complex starting 3-4 days before your vaccination appointment. Then continue to give it for several weeks afterward. (Note that fresh beef and chicken livers are a good source of B vitamins. Note also that vitamin B works better with vitamin C.)

In addition, here are some suggestions from a well known holistic veterinarian:

A good program to follow is to give pets the following vitamins beginning two to three weeks *before vaccinations, and extending two to three weeks thereafter. Vitamin A: 10,000 IU a day for a fifty pound dog, 2,500 IU a day for the adult cat. Vitamin E: dog, 400 IU a day; cat, 100 IU a day. Vitamin C: dog, 2,000 milligrams a day; cat, 500 milligrams a day. Start the C at 500 milligrams a day and increase every second day until the recommended dosage is reached. Give the dosage in stages two to three times a day. I also give a dose of 30c thuja* after vaccinating.*

— *Martin Goldstein DVM,* The Nature of Animal Healing: The Definitive Holistic Medicine Guide to Caring for Your Dog and Cat

Antioxidant Foods. Antioxidants help to destroy those troublesome free radicals we've talked about. Free radicals are atoms with unpaired electrons that mess up cells – the result of which can lead to cancer. Any injection (not just vaccinations) could cause an on-site sarcoma, due to the possible creation of free radicals. So it seems logical that foods high in antioxidants would be especially beneficial in the weeks before and after injections. Foods high in antioxidants include broccoli, cauliflower, tomatoes and peppers (use the sweet kind, not the hot, and the yellow and red rather than the green). Garlic is also good, but too much can be toxic to dogs. Some dogs love raw vegetables and some won't touch them. For the latter, simply chop up or

---

* an evergreen shrub used for homeopathic remedies

food-process the vegetables and mix them in with the pet's regular food. Or you might get creative and put ketchup on them (rich in lycopene, a good thing). There's always a way.

Stress Avoidance. Travel, a change of environment, being left in a kennel, being alone or with strangers, being adopted by new care-takers, the introduction of another animal in the house – all these can produce stress. If a pet is stressed, that's *not* the time for a shot. Try to keep your animal out of stressful situations both in the weeks before and after any vaccinations.

Exercise. Stress lowers immune systems, and exercise relieves stress. Of course a good walk every day is generally considered to be a good idea in any case – for you, too!

Nosodes. Holistic veterinarians might suggest "nosodes" to counter vaccine side effects. You can read about nosodes on page 55.

So now your furry family member is all set to be vaccinated. But it might be a *repeat* shot we're talking about – that infamous "booster" shot. Is the vaccination even *necessary?* That's what we'll look at next...

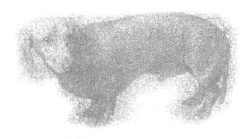

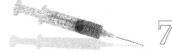

Is That Old Shot Still Working?

"You mentioned 'titer' tests. I'm not too clear on what they are. Just what does a 'titer' test?"

Titer tests are a measure of how much of a certain thing is present in a liquid. *Antibody* titers – what we're concerned with here – do one thing, and one thing *only* – they measure the amount of antibodies to a certain disease that is currently circulating in the blood. Does that mean a titer test can determine immunity to a particular disease? *Yes and no.* But first, let's see how a titer test works...

Let's say we're testing for rabies antibodies and you take a blood sample, exactly one ounce of blood. Through scientific observation you can see that there are antibodies in the

sample. You don't have to actually count them –
all you have to be able to do is to determine if
any rabies antibodies are present. Now you
discard one-half of the blood and replace it with
a dilutant. Then you test the new solution to see
if rabies antibodies are present. If they are, you
discard half of the solution again, and replace it
with the dilutant.

You keep diluting the sample in this way,
each time diluting by half and then checking for
presence of the antibodies. (This is called – what
else? – *titration*.) Your original sample (no dilution) is expressed as a 1:1 ratio. After diluting by
half, the ratio will be 1:2. Dilute again by half
and the ratio is 1:4. And so it continues: 1:8,
1:16, 1:32, etc. Sooner or later you'll get a sample
that's so diluted *no* rabies antibodies show up. So
you stop. You look at the ratio of the last sample
that showed antibodies present. It might be any-
where from 1:2 to 1:1024 (or beyond). The
number after the colon is called the titers *score*.
For example, if the last sample that showed detectable rabies antibodies was 1:16, the titers
score would be "16." Obviously, the higher the
score, the more antibodies.

HOW TITERS WORK

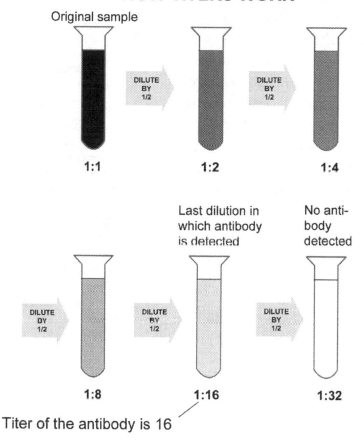

Original sample

DILUTE BY 1/2

1:1

1:2

1:4

Last dilution in which antibody is detected

No antibody detected

DILUTE BY 1/2

1:8

1:16

1:32

Titer of the antibody is 16

Many have assumed that titers can determine if an old shot is still effective; that is, if there is still immunity. But let's remember that there are other parts to the immune system other than "humoral" (meaning of the blood and

other fluids). There is also "cellular" immunity —
and this type of immunity can't be tested by
titers. There is no
simple, affordable test
for cellular immunity —
we're talking research
labs here, not routine
blood tests. Major bucks.

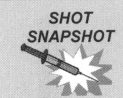

SHOT SNAPSHOT

The word "titer" is de-
rived from the French
word *titre* meaning
"title." It originally
referred to the amount
of gold or silver in a
coin.

Today, titer tests for
antibodies in the blood
are one type of several
"serological" tests.

Especially note-
worthy are the "memory
cells" we spoke of earlier.
These cells keep a
"blueprint" of a disease,
and stand ready to send
out the word to produce
antibodies to any for-
eign invaders they've
encountered in the past.
The titers may show *zero*
antibodies present in the blood, but *that doesn't
prove that immunity does not exist.*

If the body has a new exposure to the disease, the memory cells immediately go into ac-
tion, transforming themselves into "plasma"
cells, which secrete *new* antibodies against the
recognized invaders!

So what can a titer show, and what can't it
show?

Antibodies in the system will diminish over time if there is no new exposure to the disease or vaccination against it. Why should they hang around? – they know when they're not needed! But the memory cells still lurk.

So the whole complicated issue boils down to some pretty simple conclusions. And here they are:

1. If a titer shows *any* antibodies, immunity is present.
2. If a titer shows *no* antibodies, there may be immunity or there may not. If the subject has been vaccinated before, or had natural exposure, *most likely immunity is present and there is no need to revaccinate!*

From this, we can see that the only thing a titer test can absolutely indicate is: there is no need to vaccinate. It can never indicate positively the need *to* vaccinate. And remember that there is a correlation between repeated vaccinations and chronic diseases.

The American Animal Hospital Association (AAHA) in their 2006 report on Canine Vaccination Guidelines states:

Although a virus may be capable of replicating in a dog whose antibody titers have decreased, memory B and T cells should provide anamnestic (secondary) humoral and cell-mediated immune response

*that limits replication and prevents disease...
Studies...have clearly demonstrated that antibodies
to the core vaccine viruses may persist in the
absence of revaccination.*

Veterinarians also use titers to determine if a vaccination "took." (Vaccinations don't work 100% of the time.) A cautious vet may, for example, choose to give a smaller dose to your little Chihuahua than he normally gives to a Great Dane. (Many question the standard "one-size-fits-all" dose for all sizes of animals.) He may, then, do a titer as a follow-up, to make sure that the vaccine did the trick. Also, some animals just don't respond to certain vaccinations. A titer will tell.

In conclusion, I can only repeat that many, if not most, immunologists contend that any vaccination given after the first-year puppy/kitten shots – if it ever produced immunity in the first place – lasts for the life of the animal. Be very suspicious if your veterinarian tells you "Looks like Tabby needs another round of shots – just to be safe." Many recommend no vaccinations *at all* once an animal reaches adulthood, except for what is mandated by law.

"Holistic" veterinarians might even go further than that. Let's see what they are saying...

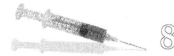

The Holistic Factor

"Some pet owners have 'holistic' veterinarians. Do these vets give shots? Or what?"

There's no absolute dividing line between veterinarians who practice traditional medicine and those who practice holistically. Many vets with conventional practices incorporate some holistic techniques and principals into their work, and *vice versa*.

Most holistic practitioners had the same training, went to the same schools of veterinary medicine and got the same basic degree ("DVM" – Doctor of Veterinary Medicine) as all the other qualified vets. Then typically at some point, they branched out into holistic, homeopathic and "alternative" fields. Holistic vets are more inclined to rely on homeopathic, herbal, and nutritional remedies, while traditional vets rely more strictly on "orthodox" medicine.

It strikes me that holistic veterinarians usually know more about traditional medicine than traditional vets know about holistic medicine, only because both received the same training in traditional veterinary basics.

As far as vaccinations are concerned, the more holistic the practitioner, I find, the more that vaccines are totally shunned. Conversely, the traditional purist will tend to trust more in vaccines and totally discredit holistic methods of disease prevention. Most vets, I would venture, fall between these extremes.

Part of the case against holism is the fact that holistic remedies are much more difficult to scientifically evaluate. For many technical reasons, it's just harder to test holistic methods. Also, with drug corporations having little interest in the outcomes of holistic tests, there is less financial backing for significant studies.

So – much of the evidence for holism is anecdotal. Nevertheless, holistic veterinarians testify to significant successes in their own practices – and these are hard to deny. If a vet sees the same remedy working again and again over many years, that simply can't be discounted. As the old saw goes, "It's hard to argue with success."

Dr. Richard H. Pitcairn, a noted holistic author, acknowledges the differences of opinion regarding vaccinations in the animal health community. Here he is addressing the issue of vaccinating cats ill with feline immunodeficiency virus (sometimes called feline AIDS) or other viral disease:

> *Another important point is that any cat suspected of having FIV (or feline leukemia or other chronic viruses) should never be vaccinated. That's because the vaccine viruses stress the body (possibly triggering the latent state) and depress the immune system in many cats (again allowing the virus to get started). The principle is to avoid anything that will disturb or weaken the immune system. I know this advice runs counter to that of many veterinarians, who encourage vaccination as a way to protect a weakened cat. My clinical experience and background in immunology, however, convince me that this is the worst thing to do.*
>
> *– Richard H. Pitcairn and Susan Hubble Pitcairn,* Dr. Pitcairn's New Complete Guide to Natural Health for Dogs and Cats

Dr. Pitcairn is virtually saying "What am I to believe – convention? or my own experience?"

Nosodes

Some holistic veterinarians completely reject vaccinations and rely instead on "nosodes," which are preparations typically given orally, not injected. The word "nosode" comes from the

Greek word *nosos*, simply meaning "disease." To understand what a nosode is, you have to know a little about homeopathy, since nosodes are homeopathic alternatives to vaccines.

Homeopathy, if I may oversimplify, is the making and administering of remedies made from substances derived from or similar to the disease being treated.

There are two classes of materials used. The first includes derivatives from plants, minerals and animals – the general natural world. The second (here it gets a little distasteful sounding), from diseased tissue, mucus, pus, discharges and cultures of microorganisms. The substances are diluted and diluted, to the point where they are harmless and barely detectable in the solution. There are specific standards for exactly the amount of dilution for each remedy. The principle of "less is more" applies, according to homeopathic practice.

The preparation is then given by mouth. The theory is an old one, that of pitting "like" against "like," going back a couple of centuries. Homeopathic remedies are considered to be safe, and have virtually no side effects.

Now about those nosodes. These are preparations usually made from the second class of substances – those derived from sick animals and even people. The diseased material is diluted until it is harmless.

Every nosode is associated with a certain disease. For example, there's a nosode for rabies, one for distemper, etc.

Do nosodes work? Do they provide immunity? There are no conclusive studies proving that they give reliable protection. There is, however, some evidence that they work in the case of epidemics. There are documented cases showing that groups given nosodes have less incidence of disease during epidemics. In an outbreak of meningitis in Brazil in 1974, over 18,000 children were given nosodes against the disease. They fared 8

SHOT SNAPSHOT

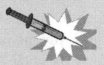

Nosodes and the Law

If you decide to go the nosode route, keep in mind that nosodes do not generally fulfill legal requirements for vaccination.

Most kennels requiring vaccinations and international customs agents do not accept nosodes as meeting vaccination requirements.

States mandating rabies vaccinations, however, may waive requirements if the animal is ill and therefore not a candidate for vaccines. In this case, a pet owner may turn to a rabies nosode.

times better than children who were not given nosodes. There are other such examples showing favorable results in outbreaks of other diseases as well.

But – and this is a big but – there are no studies to suggest that nosodes give *lasting* protection. Anyone depending solely on nosodes had better talk with their veterinarian about periodically repeating them.

Nosodes do *not* produce antibodies. That is often given as a reason for their lack of providing immunity. This, however, misses the whole point, say homeopaths. They would tell you that nosodes provide an entirely different kind of immunity, that they act on another, deeper level than antibody based immunity, reducing the body's *sensitivity* to viral and bacterial invaders.

So what's the bottom line? All I can do is throw out some ideas for you to consider, and let you decide.

1. If you completely reject traditional vaccines, then nosodes make perfect sense, since they will do no harm.
2. If you choose to vaccinate (judiciously), and want extra protection, then consider nosodes in a supplemental role.

3. Nosodes can help if used before –
and after – vaccinations. Holists
suggest that they help the immune
system withstand the vaccines.

4. Nosodes are safe to use in puppies
and kittens as young as three weeks
old.

5. Nosodes could play a role as re-
placements for "booster" vaccinations in previously vaccinated animals in cases where you're not feeling sure about revaccinating.

6. Vaccinations just don't work with
some animals, as revealed in titer
tests. Nosodes might then be the
only alternative.

7. If your pet is suffering from a bad
vaccination response ("vaccinosis"),
nosodes may help to reduce the ill
effects.

As you have seen, there are many opinions
from the experts. What I'd like to do now is tell
you how some of our major veterinary insti-
tutions weigh in on all this...

Group-Speak:
Official Recommendations

"You've expressed your opinions and related quite a few opinions of others. What I'd like to hear is something more, well, *authoritative*. What's the *consensus* on vaccinations?"

There are three principal organizations that sponsor studies and report on recent findings regarding veterinary vaccines. These are the American Animal Hospital Association (AAHA), the American Veterinary Medical Association (AVMA), and the American Association of Feline Practitioners (AAFP). All three publish "guidelines" reflecting the current thinking and findings in their respective veterinary communities.

Many university schools of veterinary medicine also publish detailed guidelines and recommendations regarding canine and feline vaccines. Since much of this material is based upon the three groups mentioned above, and a lot of the information overlaps, we'll not go into the university publications here. You will find the Web sites of several of these veterinary schools listed in the Resources pages at the end of this book, should you want to explore further.

American Animal Hospital Association

The AAHA's Canine Vaccine Task Force published Canine Vaccination Guidelines in 2003, and again in 2006. While the AAHA is rooted basically in conventional medicine only, their work is quite comprehensive and their recommendations are detailed and specific. Their guidelines are divided into two groups – guidelines for general veterinary practice and guidelines for shelters. In this book we'll concern ourselves only with the general guidelines.

You won't find much support for holistic ideas in the AAHA papers, as evidenced in the following excerpt from their 2003 guidelines:

> *Do Not Use Nosodes (Holistic Vaccines) to vaccinate a puppy. Nosodes do not provide immunity; thus, the puppy will remain susceptible to the disease the nosode was designed to prevent.*

Use a USDA-licensed vaccine to immunize puppies.

This warning refers only to puppies, and no opinion is subsequently given on using nosodes on adult dogs, so they leave room here for some friendliness (or at least ambivalence) towards holism. Their 2006 Guidelines concur with much of the opinion expressed in this book regarding the limiting of needless vaccinations.

The AAHA report classifies vaccines as *core, non-core,* and *non-recommended.* Core vaccines are those which are generally recommended for all dogs. Non-core vaccines are optional, to be evaluated according to environmental, lifestyle, and individual medical concerns. Nonrecommended vaccines are those unapproved because they are considered either ineffective or unsafe.

What is abundantly clear in the AAHA Guidelines is the emphasis on the need to consider each patient individually. They stress again and again that veterinarians should construct vaccination plans according to the breed, age, and general medical profile of their patients.

The AAHA 2006 report lists the following as **Core Vaccines for dogs** –

Canine Parvovirus (Modified Live Virus)
Canine Distemper (MLV)

*r*Canine Distemper
Canine Adenovirus-2 (MLV parenteral)
Rabies 1-year (killed)
Rabies 3-year (killed)

Here are the **Non-core Vaccines for dogs** –

Distemper Measles Virus
Parainfluenza Virus (MLV-parenteral)
Bordetella bronchiseptica (killed bacterin) – parenteral
Bordetella bronchiseptica (live avirulent bacteria) + Parainfluenza Virus (MLV) – topical (intra-nasal) application
Bordetella bronchiseptica (cell wall antigen extract) – parenteral
Borrelia burgdorferi (Lyme borreliosis) (killed whole bacterin) or Borrelia burgdorferi (rLyme borreliosis) (recombinant-Outer surface protein A [OspA])
Leptospira interrogans (combined with serovars canicola and icterohaemorrhagiae) (killed bacterin)

The following are **Not Recommended for dogs** –

Canine Parvovirus (killed)
Canine Adenovirus-1 (MLV and killed)
Canine Adenovirus-2 (killed or MLV topical)
Canine Coronavirus (killed and MLV)
Giardia lamblia (killed)

Looking at the "Not Recommended" list, above, you may wonder why the AAHA is not recommending the *killed* version of Parvovirus while recommending the Modified *Live* Virus version of this vaccine. Aren't killed-virus vaccines safer than live-virus ones?

Well, not always. Sometimes the killed version just doesn't do the trick of providing solid protection. In the case of Parvo, puppies might need many doses of the killed version, due to "maternal antibody interference." Simply put, this means that the body is putting up a resistance.

So one good dose of the (modified) *live* vaccine offers much better protection. This particular vaccine offers a duration of immunity (DOI) of seven years – a much better choice. In spite of this AAHA recommendation, though, one might still worry about the adverse effects live vaccines have been known to cause.

On the *other* hand, Jean Dodds, whose advice we observed on page 38, specifies "MLV" for her Parvo, so there's some solid advice out there urging the live virus shot. I never promised you that all the advice printed in this book would be consistent. My personal advice? Go with the *live* on the Parvo.

Notice on the "core" list that there are two versions of Canine Distemper vaccines. The *live* (MLV) vaccine has traditionally been the only one available. Now there is an alternate version in the one with the little "r" in front, meaning "recombinant."

What's *that* all about? Read the following inset about one recombinant type of vaccine:

SHOT SNAPSHOT

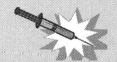

Live Vectored Vaccines

A live vectored vaccine is made by using yeast or bacteria to make large quantities of a protein of the virus or bacteria that causes the disease. When this protein is injected into the body, the immune system makes antibodies to the disease agent's protein.

This creates an immunity to the disease from which the protein was made, without actually introducing the disease itself into the body.

There is zero chance of getting the disease from a live vectored vaccine, since the actual virus or bacteria aren't introduced into the body. Another advantage is that live vectored vaccines don't need adjuvants, which are suspected of causing adverse results (such as cancer).

If I had my druthers, I'd certainly take the "recombinant" version over the live virus version. The AAHA writes:

*r*Canine Distemper:
A suitable alternative to the MLV Canine Distemper Virus and may be used interchangeably with the MLV-CDV vaccine. Recent unpublished studies have shown that compared with the MLV-CDV vaccines, the recombinant CDV vaccine is more likely to immunize puppies in the face of Passively Acquired Maternal Antibody (PAMA).

"*Suitable alternative*??" Why not "*Way better* alternative?" More likely to immunize? No cancer-causing adjuvants? No chance of getting the disease from the vaccine?

When I heard about recombinants, my first thought was to hire a skywriter and emblazon the message across the heavens. Let's just say, for my money, they're a no-brainer.

By the way, you may be wondering what "passively acquired maternal antibodies" are. These (PAMA) are antibodies that have been passed down to the young animal from the mother. They can interfere with immunization from vaccines and cause "antigenic intolerance" – a condition in which vaccines are rendered ineffective by the body.

Need more info? The AAHA 2006 Guidelines are quite detailed. The complete report is available online at:

www.aahanet.org/About_aaha/About_Position.html

American Veterinary Medical Association

The AVMA is the leading organization of veterinarians in the United States – the "AMA" of the veterinary world. On their Web site they present information for pet owners, as well as veterinary health professionals. The Association gives their positions and policies on all things veterinary, and there is much written on vaccines, as one might expect. Here are some of the highlights:

"Is it important to vaccinate?" is one of the first questions posed. The answer, in part:

> Yes! Pets should be vaccinated to protect them from many highly contagious and deadly diseases. Experts agree that widespread use of vaccines within the last century has prevented death and disease in millions of animals. Even though some formerly common diseases have now become uncommon, vaccination is still highly recommended because these serious disease agents continue to be present in the environment.

The question of whether vaccines ensure protection for your pet is answered in this way:

> For most pets, vaccination is effective and will prevent future disease. Occasionally, a vaccinated pet may not develop adequate immunity and, although rare, it is possible for these pets to become ill. It is important to remember that although breakdowns in protection do occur, most successfully vaccinated pets never show signs of disease, making vaccination an important part of your pet's preventive health care.

Remember that a titer test given a few weeks after vaccination will determine whether or not immunity was achieved. Without this check, you'll never really know if your animal is immunized or not. I note that "signs of disease" refers to the disease the pet is being vaccinated against, not diseases the vaccine might cause ("adverse responses"). The question of risks is addressed thusly:

Although most pets respond well to vaccines, like any medical procedure vaccination carries some risk. The most common adverse responses are mild and short-term, including fever, sluggishness, and reduced appetite. Pets may also experience temporary pain or subtle swelling at the site of vaccination. Although most adverse responses will resolve within a day or two, excessive pain, swelling, or listlessness should be discussed with your veterinarian.

Rarely, serious adverse responses occur. Contact your veterinarian immediately if your pet has repeated vomiting or diarrhea, whole body itching, difficulty breathing, collapse, or swelling of the face or legs. These signs may indicate an allergic reaction. In very rare instances death can occur. Visit with your veterinarian about the latest information on vaccine safety, including rare adverse responses that may develop weeks or months after vaccination.

The problem with "rare adverse responses," as I see it is that the adverse effects that appear months or years later usually aren't (or can't be) attributed to the vaccination that caused them. As to the question of limiting the number and types of vaccinations, the AVMA advises:

> *Discuss with your veterinarian your pet's lifestyle, access to other animals, and travel to other geographic locations, since these factors affect your pet's risk of exposure to disease. Not all pets should be vaccinated with all vaccines just because these vaccines are available.*

I would guess that one of the biggest mistakes pet owners make is not heeding the advice in that last sentence.

As to the duration of immunity (DOI) offered by vaccines, the Association allows that "there is increasing evidence that immunity triggered by some vaccines provides protection beyond one year." Compared to other authoritative sources, I find this much too cautious a statement, considering that some respected experts attest that many vaccinations last "three years," "seven years" and even "for the life of the animal" in some cases. The only further advice given on the subject is to "talk with your veterinarian about what is best for your pet."

For more information, check out:

www.avma.org/careforanimals/animatedjourneys/pethealth/vaccinations.asp

and
www.avma.org/issues/policy/vaccination_principles.asp

American Association of Feline Practitioners

The AAFP and the Academy of Feline Medicine Advisory Panel on Feline Vaccines issued a 28-page report in 2000. The report (their most recent) is directed to veterinarians to use as a guide in their vaccination practices.

The AAFP doesn't use the "core" and "non-core" classifications, just a simple "highly recommended," "routine use of this vaccine is not recommended," or "not recommended." The Association seems to be aware of the dangers of over-vaccinating as well as the fact that vaccines aren't bulletproof:

In the introduction, the report states that "most vaccines do not induce complete protection from infection or disease, nor do they induce the same degree of protection in all animals."

The general position on vaccinations seems to be pretty well summed up in this paragraph (emphasis is mine):

The overall objectives of vaccination are to vaccinate the largest possible number of individuals in the population at risk, vaccinate each individual <u>no more frequently than necessary</u>, and vaccinate <u>only against infectious agents to which individuals</u>

have a realistic risk of exposure and subsequent development of disease.

The distinction between kittens and adults, and how each should be approached is made clear:

> _Kittens younger than 16 weeks of age are generally more susceptible to infection than are adult cats and typically develop more severe disease. Thus, they represent the principal target population for vaccination. Maternal antibody interference is the most common reason why some animals are not immunized following vaccination, and is the reason why a series of vaccinations is necessary for kittens younger than 12 weeks of age. Vaccination needs of adult cats should be assessed at least once yearly, and if necessary, modified on the basis of an assessment of their risk._

Highly Recommended Vaccines –

Here then, are the vaccines designated as "Highly Recommended:"

Feline panleukopenia (Feline parvovirus – FPV). Clinical signs of feline panleukopenia (commonly called distemper) include lethargy, anorexia, vomiting, diarrhea, and abnormally low white blood cell count.

"[Certain data] indicate that a parenteral* FPV vaccine induces immunity for at least 7 years. Recommendation on repeat shots: After initial series and revaccination one year later, repeat shots no more frequently than every 3 years." It is suggested that the feline parvovirus vaccine also protects cats against the canine form of parvo. Caution: Don't vaccinate pregnant females or kittens less that 1 month old.

Feline viral rhinotracheitis and feline calcivirus infection (FHV-1 and FCV). Risk of exposure is high, since this respiratory disease is widespread in the feline population. Kittens are especially at risk, while the disease is rarely serious in adult cats. Protection lasts "at least 3 years." Caution: avoid vaccinating kittens younger than 4 weeks of age with modified live virus version.

Rabies. More cats than dogs develop rabies in the United States. Recommendations: "Treatment is ineffective in cats that develop clinical signs, and should not be attempted." Problems: Vaccine-associated sarcomas are reported, however such sarcomas are more frequently associated with feline leukemia virus.

Special note: The feline rabies vaccine comes in three flavors: Adjuvenated inactivated-

---

* introduced otherwise than by way of the intestines (such as by injection)

virus vaccine for parenteral administration every year, Adjuvenated inactivated-virus vaccine for parenteral administration every *three* years, and Canarypox virus-vectored *recombinant* vaccine for parenteral administration.

[Personally, I would go with the recombinant, since it lacks an adjuvant. However, it's recommended that the recombinant version be repeated every year, as opposed to the three-year version. If local laws mandate rabies shots every year, then, in my opinion, the recombinant version is the obvious choice.]

Vaccines Not Routinely Recommended –

The following basically fall under the heading "Routine use of this vaccine is not recommended." (This is not to say that the vaccine is *never* recommended, rather that certain risk factors should be considered before its use.)

Feline leukemia virus infection (FeLV). The signs of this disease are related to neoplasia (tumors), anemia, and immunosuppressive disorders. Outdoor cats and those living in multiple-cat situations are most at risk. The virus is typically transmitted directly from cat to cat, or from sharing food and water utensils.

Kittens are more susceptible to infection than older cats, since resistance grows as cats mature. The report advises that the decision to vaccinate against feline leukemia should be based on the animal's age and the risk of exposure. If your cat lives in a closed, feline leukemia-negative environment and is over 4 months of age, there is little risk of developing the disease.

Special note: Studies vary as to the efficacy of this vaccine. The report states, *"Because protection is not induced in all [vaccinated cats], preventing exposure to infected cats remains the single best way to prevent FeLV infection."* [italics in original]

Chlamydiosis – *Chlamydia psittaci.* The most common sign of this disease is conjunctivitis (an eye inflammation sometimes called "pinkeye.") The report basically states that the signs of the disease are usually mild and easy to treat, and the vaccine is associated with greater concerns for "adverse events." It is suggested that you might consider using the vaccine for situations in which infection is present in multiple-cat environments.

Dermatophytosis. This is primarily an infection with *Microsporum canis*, a fungus that causes lesions on the skin – a "ringworm" in cats. At the time of the report (2000) the vaccine had not been evaluated for efficacy, and so was not recommended. [There are several effective treatments for ringworm in cats, and the disease is self-limiting. The report advises considering the vaccine only if there is an outbreak in a multiple-cat environment.]

Bordetella bronchiseptica infection. Bordetella is a disease of the respiratory tract found in cats, dogs ("kennel cough"), and several other animals. It is thought to be transmitted through the air, from one animal to another. Signs include sneezing, coughing, and fever. Again, here is a disease that can be cured with treatment, hence the "not routinely recommended" categorization. At the time of the report, the efficacy of the recently released vaccine had not been evaluated in multiple-cat environments.

Giardiasis – Giardia lamblia. This is a gastrointestinal disease that can range from mild to severe. The disease is transmitted from fecal material directly by mouth, and by contaminated water. A cat can also acquire the disease from grooming another cat that's been infected. At the time of the report, the vaccine had not been independently evaluated, although it had been approved for cats 8 weeks of age or older.

Not Recommended –

One vaccine was not recommended for use:

   Feline infectious peritonitis (FIP).
There are two groups of feline coronavirus disease. There is a mild form called "enteric" coronavirus (FECV) that is generally not a problem
to treat. However, FECV, it is believed, can
mutate into feline infectious peritonitis viruses
(FIPV), and these can cause feline infectious
peritonitis (FIP). About 1-5% of cats with feline
coronavirus will ultimately develop FIP (mostly
kittens).
   The ability of the FIP vaccine to prevent
disease is surrounded by controversy, with some
studies showing protection, others not. The
Association does not recommend the vaccine,
stating that *"at this time, there is no evidence
that the vaccine induces clinically relevant
protection."*

———————

   Finally, a note regarding "administration
sites" (where on the cat's body to give injections
of which vaccines). The following guidelines are
quoted in their entirety from the AAFP report:

   ▶ *Vaccines containing antigens limited to
      feline parvovirus, feline herpesvirus-1, and*

feline calcivirus (with or without Chlamydia psittaci) should be administered over the <u>right shoulder</u> (avoiding midline), as distally[*] as possible.

▶ *Vaccines containing rabies virus antigen (plus any other antigen) should be administered on the <u>right rear limb</u>, as distally as possible*

▶ *Vaccines containing feline leukemia virus antigen (plus any other antigen except rabies virus antigen) should be administered on the <u>left rear limb</u>, as distally as possible.*

▶ *Injection sites of other medications should be recorded.*

The complete report can be found online:

www.aafponline.org/resources/guidelines/vaccine.pdf

So much for studies, trends and group opinions and conclusions. How about hearing from individual veterinarians? That's next...

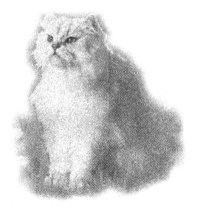

---

[*] far away from the center of the body

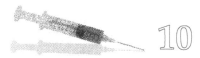

10

General Advice From Veterinarians

"Do veterinarians agree with the official vaccine guidelines? Or do they have other opinions based on their own experience?"

In addition to reading the opinions expressed in institutional reports of the major veterinary associations, it's valuable to find out what individual veterinarians are thinking. After all, they're the ones down there "in the trenches" observing the effects of vaccines firsthand.

For this chapter, I'm going to just sit back and let their words speak for themselves. Most of these comments are from vets of the holistic persuasion. That's not because I want to slant things in their direction – holistic vets just seem to write more than traditional ones. And here they provide balance to the previous chapter, which mostly covers the orthodox view.

Gary Van Engelenburg, DVM. Sparky and I were guests on a TV show a few years ago along with Gary Van Engelenburg, DVM, a knowledgeable holistic veterinarian from Des Moines, Iowa. While writing this book I thought he might have an opinion regarding pet vaccinations, and, sure enough, he did:

"The annual vaccine habit wouldn't be so bad if it was as simple as not being necessary. The truth is that there are harmful side effects to giving MLV (modified live virus) vaccines every year. More and more research in this area is coming up with the vaccines causing auto-immune antibody production to many organs and body tissues. When you consider that immune titers studies indicate a minimum of 7 years protection after a single dose where do we get the annual booster idea anyway? I think we, as veterinarians, are obligated to do what is best for the pet. Giving unnecessary vaccines, in my opinion, is unethical and, in some instances, bordering on malpractice.

"Another factor to consider is safety when giving MLV vaccines, especially when giving multiple antigens at the same time. Most of our continuing education on new vaccines and vaccine combinations comes from representatives of the companies selling the product. I can't help but think there may be a bit of bias involved here. Anyway, we are constantly told that the multiple antigen products are safe, convenient and effective.

"I remember two cases in the past year with perfectly normal, happy, apparently healthy cats being presented in complete total flaccid paralysis within 72 hours after getting 'all their shots.' Extensive diagnostics had been done on both animals by their regular vet before being presented to me and in both cases the owners were told that nothing was apparently wrong with their pet and that the vaccines couldn't be at fault!!! Many times every month I hear new clients complain about their pet being sick for up to 2 weeks after receiving multiple vaccines at once. I think our own pets are telling us something and maybe we should listen to them."

Donna Kelleher, DVM: Here's what this veterinarian writes in her book "The Last Chance Dog (2004):

"Whenever you are trying to make decisions as to whether to vaccinate your pet, you must weigh the risk versus benefit. In other words, if your dog is young, say under three years old, vaccines might really benefit him. If he is older, especially if he is not well, the risks may outweigh the benefits. Other factors include travel history, exposure to wildlife, and, especially, contact with other dogs and parasites that may put your pet more at risk."

Donald Hamilton, DVM: In his highly regarded book "Homeopathic Care for Cats and Dogs," (1999) this doctor writes about the conflicts between animal vaccination laws and the lack of medical necessity to have them:

"I recognize that, since most state laws require rabies vaccines, this creates a difficult crossroad. I can only recommend here that you fight to change the laws in your state. As a veterinarian, I am obligated to uphold rabies vaccination laws, thus I cannot recommend refusing rabies vaccination. If you contemplate avoiding rabies vaccination for your companion, you must realize that this is a legal decision as well as a medical decision. Rabies vaccines typically provide lifetime immunity, at least after two doses, so the need for further vaccination is legal, not medical...With few exceptions (some communities may require other vaccines though no state law requires them, to my knowledge), all other vaccines are optional. I recommend avoiding vaccination in almost all circumstances, as I believe it mainly creates illness rather than preventing illness."

Some Quick Quotables: The following quotes appeared in a survey about vaccinations in *Wolf Clan Magazine* (now defunct), in its April-May 1995 (!) issue:

I believe that poor diet and vaccinations are responsible for most chronic diseases.
                    – Russell Swift, DVM, Tamarac, FL

The first thing that must change with routine vaccinations is the myth that vaccines are not harmful. Veterinarians and animal guardians have to come to realize that they are not protecting animals from disease by annual vaccinations, but in fact, are destroying the health and immune systems of these same animals they love and care for.
                    – Charles E. Loops, DVM, Pittsboro, NC

Vaccinosis is the reaction from common inoculations (vaccines) against the body's immune system and general well-being. These reactions might take months or years to show up and will cause undue harm to future generations.
                    – Pedro Rivera, DVM BS, Harrisburg, PA

The most common problems I see that are directly related to vaccines on a day to day basis are ear or skin conditions, such as chronic discharges and itching. I also see behavior problems such as fearfulness or aggression.
                    – Pat Bradley, DVM, Conway, AR

Routine vaccinations are probably the worst thing that we do for our animals... Repeating vaccinations on a yearly basis undermines the whole energetic well-being of our animals.

— Christina Chambreau, DVM, Sparks, MD

There are a lot of chronic conditions that [can] develop some time after vaccinating. Some of these conditions that I see are chronic ear infections, digestive problems, seizures, skin problems, and behavioral problems.

— Stephen Blake, DVM, CVH CVA
San Diego, CA

Unfortunately our society is in the grasp of a health panacea and this panacea is fuelled by the bio-medical and pharmaceutical industries. Vaccinations have become the modern day equivalent of leeching.

— Mike Kohn, DVM, Madison, WI

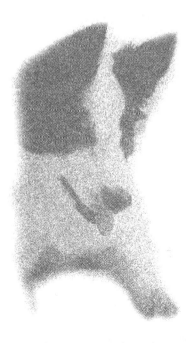

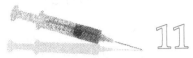

Vaccination Do's and Don'ts

"I've read up to here, but I'm not sure just where to start, or how to apply all this information. Could you sort of boil it all down?"

Every pet owner can't be expected to make the expert judgments of an immunologist, or know all there is to know. All I've tried to do in these few pages is to send out a wakeup call on the dangers. Many animal caretakers already have an appreciation of what I'm saying here but, I would venture, these are in the minority. I'm simply trying to change that.

If everyone knew just a few basics, it would go a long way towards saving more of our furry friends' lives. Vaccinations, as we have seen, are suspected of being a leading trigger of cancer, allergies, and various autoimmune diseases in dogs and cats. If everyone would just become aware that those annual booster shots lower the immune system, and in the case of young puppies, over-vaccinating can do permanent damage, and some of the other ways in which shots can carry threats as well as protections, then this book would be no longer needed. *And I hope that's what happens!*

So here is my personal list of "do's and don'ts." If you take away nothing else from this book, I suggest you absorb what follows:

DO educate yourself about the risks of vaccinating, as compared to the benefits, so that you can make intelligent decisions. If you are reading this book you've already begun to inform yourself.

DO make your veterinarian aware of your concerns about the dangers of vaccinations. For each injection, ask exactly what it is for and if it is really necessary. If your vet is aware of your concerns, he or she is less likely to over-vaccinate. Remember that 50% of the practices of most veterinarians is in giving shots. A veterinarian may well be ethical, but is not financially motivated to limit vaccinations. That $80 vaccination visit may have cost the vet $5-$10 for the vaccine.

DO (if you choose to vaccinate) restrict vaccinations to diseases endemic in your area and your pet's activities. For example, if your dog won't be in a region where Lyme disease is a risk, omit Lyme disease vaccinations. If your pet won't be boarded with others, you may omit Bordetella shots, etc.

DO keep records of each vaccination, what was given and on what date. When acquiring a new dog or cat make sure to get records from previous caretakers!

DO know your local laws about canine and feline vaccinations. Most areas require only rabies shots. Some localities (misguided, in my opinion) mandate other shots as well.

DO ask for a "titer" test if there is any question about the necessity for a booster shot. Most shots typically given to one-year-olds and older last longer than one year, and many much longer, possibly for the life or the pet. Automatic "annual boosters" should be avoided!

DO remember that titer tests never prove that a revaccination is needed, no matter how low the titers score. A titer counts anti-bodies present in the blood. These tests can only show when a vaccination is *not* needed. If *any* antibodies are detected, no vaccination is necessary. If *none* are detected, this alone does not prove the necessity for a revaccination (although some might suggest otherwise).

DO prepare your animal for shots by boosting the immune system before and after inoculations. Ask your vet about giving your pet daily Vitamin B Complex and other supplements (see page 44) for several days before and a few weeks after receiving vaccines. (Vitamin C helps the B to work better.) Consider using nosodes, as recommended on page 46.

DO be aware that "modified live virus" (MLV) vaccines can carry more risk of becoming virulent than "killed" virus vaccines. On the other hand, killed versions usually contain more (dangerous) adjuvants. Ask your vet if the vaccines to be given are live or killed. Discuss the risks and benefits of each alternative. (I would also ask if a recombinant version is available!)

DO (if you choose *not* to vaccinate) comensate by boosting the immune system using nutritional, herbal and holistic means.

DON'T over-vaccinate a newly acquired puppy or kitten. Oftentimes the breeder or shelter has already vaccinated the animal, and the new owner repeats the same vaccinations. Remember that vaccinations lower the immune system, inviting cancer and other diseases to take hold. Note that if immunity exists, revaccinating doesn't add to the immunity. Be especially careful about repeating live virus vaccines. The worst effects of over-vaccinating may not show up right away; it may be years – but they will show up!

DON'T give vaccinations close to periods when your cat or dog will undergo stress. If you are going on vacation and plan on kenneling your dog while you're away, give kennel cough shots (or whatever) several weeks in advance. Stress and vaccinations each lower the immune system. Asking a poor animal to handle them both at the same time is never a good idea. With new adoptions, wait until they have overcome the stress of dealing with their new environment before giving shots.

DON'T give more than one vaccination at a time! This is especially true in the case of puppies and kittens. Allow at least three weeks between vaccinations. And for rabies shots, separate from other vaccines by at least a full month before and after. When possible, avoid "combination" or "multivalent" vaccines (typically three or more diseases mixed up in one "cocktail.") There is no absolute proof that these multi-shots are dangerous, but why take the chance if you don't have to? Sometimes they are unavoidable, since some vaccines aren't available singly – only in these multivalents!

DON'T give a rabies shot to a puppy or kitten until he/she is six months old. Laws sometimes mandate giving rabies shots at three months – try to prolong this if you can. Most professionals agree that puppies' and kittens' immune systems aren't well enough developed at three months.

DON'T give shots for diseases that are easily curable (with antibiotics or other means). Many find that it's easier, for example, to deal with curing corona (a viral intestinal infection of dogs) than the side effects of the vaccine.

DON'T expose other pets to a pet that has received "live" virus shots for 10-21 days after receiving the shots. Live vaccines "shed" through the skin and feces, and could be dangerous to other dogs and cats.

DON'T vaccinate a sick animal or an adult female during seasons, when hormonal changes are taking place.

Finally, I would hope that you, knowing what you now know, would be concerned about pets other than your own, and help spread the word to other dog or cat owners like yourself. There are *millions* of dogs and *millions* of cats in The United States alone. Let's give them a break. Let's not let them become the victims of over-vaccinating. Let's help dispel the idea that vaccinations are panaceas, with no down sides.

Now that you know the real dangers of over-vaccinating, beware! Use your head. When they don't make sense, *Stop The Shots!*

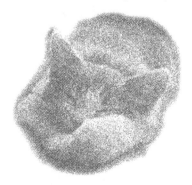

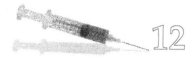

On The Horizon

"I'm curious about the future and new developments. What are the scientists working on that might advance the practice of animal vaccinations?"

Medical advances seem to be popping up at exponentially faster rates every day, and the field of veterinary vaccines is no exception. Here are a few of the new technologies that you might find one of these days "at a vet near you."

Up to now the two main types of vaccines consisted of viruses or bacteria that are either "killed" or "modified live." But there are new approaches being developed that go beyond the concept of using whole microorganisms of the disease itself combined with adjuvants.

Some or these – "live vectored" vaccines and "subunit" vaccines are already available. Others are under investigation, such as "gene-deleted" vaccines and vaccines made only of Deoxyribonucleic acid (DNA).

New adjuvants (ingredients to enhance the immune system response) are also being developed. The goals are to make vaccines safer and more effective, and the work focuses on diseases for which vaccines already exist as well as diseases for which no successful vaccines have been produced as yet.

Here, in brief, are a few of the "cutting edge" developments:

Live Vectored Vaccines (see "recombinant" vaccine on page 65) are made from proteins that are caused to be produced by a virus, not the virus itself. The advantage is that, since the virus isn't actually introduced into the body, there is no chance of virulence that might cause the disease. Live vectored vaccines don't need adjuvants, another plus. This type of vaccine is already available for canine distemper. Since this vaccine contains genes only from distemper and not the entire virus genome, there's no chance a dog can get distemper from the shot. This type of vaccine also overcomes possible resistance to immunization caused by maternal antibodies. I think we will be hearing more about live vectored vaccines being developed for other canine and feline diseases!

Gene-Deleted Vaccines. These are not available for pet animals, but seem promising. Researchers in Japan, for instance, reported a gene-deleted vaccine that immunized monkeys against HIV infection. The idea is basically to take a virus, alter or remove one of its genes, and make a killed or modified live vaccine from it. The "deleted" gene has to be one that is "non-required" in order for the vaccine to produce immunity. The advantage of these vaccines is non-virulence, hence a safer shot. Stay tuned.

Sub-unit Vaccines. The idea behind this one is "Why use the whole virus, when you only have to use that part of the virus that's needed to produce immunity?" These vaccines contain only a portion of the organism that would be used in a conventional vaccine. Since irrelevant proteins are not used, you don't need as much vaccine to do the trick, an advantage. The disadvantage is that for some diseases you need more than one protein to produce protection. Sub-unit vaccines therefore seem limited. Encouragingly, there was a Lyme disease subunit vaccine that showed promising results when recently tested on dogs in an area where Lyme disease is endemic.

DNA (Deoxyribonucleic Acid) Vaccines. We hear so much these days about DNA, especially in the field of criminal investigations, where DNA samples are used to prove or disprove identity. It seems odd to see the term "DNA" turn up in the field of immunology. But when you think about it, it makes perfect sense.

What, ultimately, produces disease fighting antibodies? Not the virus or bacterial content of the vaccine. What produces antibodies are the *antigens* stimulated by these microorganisms. What if you could produce the antigens *without* using the actual virus – do an end run around the virus itself? What if you could directly introduce into the body the *genetic coding* for the antigens? *Presto! – antibodies!* That's what DNA vaccines are all about.

This is about as exciting as immunology gets. So far, however, there are no DNA vaccines for dogs and cats, although one for West Nile virus has been recently licensed for horses. The vaccines, by the way, aren't administered by the typical hypodermic needle method into the bloodstream, since the DNA has to get into the host cells. In addition to needle injection directly into the muscle, there are special no-needle injectors to get the DNA through the skin as well as "gene guns" that shoot gold microbeads with the DNA on them into the body. (This method gives "shot" a whole new meaning!)

There are potentially many advantages to this technology: overcoming maternal antibody interference, duration of immunity (unlimited?), affordability(!), stability – and the possibility of eliminating the downside of vaccines altogether!!

Perhaps one day vaccinations will be 100% safe. 100% effective.

Perhaps one day there will be no need for a book such as this! Until then – take care, stay educated, and approach the currently available technology with an inquiring, discriminating eye!

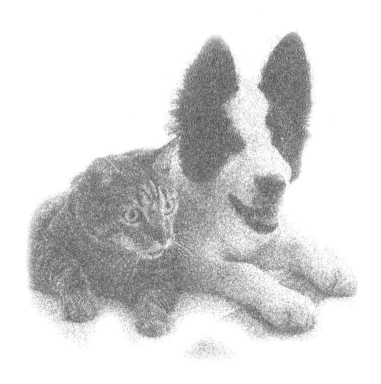

Resources

BOOKS

277 Secrets Your Cat Wants You to Know; Paulette Cooper, Paul Noble (1997)

Business Basics for Veterinarians; Lowell Ackerman (2002)

Canine Medicine and Disease Prevention; S. Mario Durrant, Jane Fishman Leon, Cody W. Faerber, (2004)

Complete Book of Dog Breeding, The; Dan Rice (1996)

Complete Holistic Dog Book: Home Health Care for Our Canine Companions; Katy Sommers Allegretti (2003)

Complete Idiot's Guide to Dog Health and Nutrition, The; Margaret H. Bonham, Jim Wingert (2003)

Dr. Pitcairn's New Complete Guide to Natural Health for Dogs and Cats; Richard H. Pitcairn and Susan Hubble (2005)

Encyclopedia of Natural Pet Care, The; C. J. Puotinen (2000)

Everything Small Dogs Book; Kathy Salzberg (2005)

Everything You Need to Know About Lyme Disease; Karen Donnelly (2000)

Feline Medicine And Disease Management; S. Mario Durrant, Jane Fishman Leon, Cody W. Faerber, (2005)

Holistic Guide For A Healthy Dog, The; Wendy Volhard, Kerry Brown (1995)

Holistic Puppy, The: How to Have a Happy, Healthy Dog; Diane Stein (1998)

Homeopathic Care for Cats and Dogs; Donald Hamilton (1999)

Last Chance Dog, The: And Other True Stories of Holistic Animal Healing; Donna Kelleher (2004)

Natural Healing for Dogs and Cats; Diane Stein (1993)

Natural Remedy Book for Dogs & Cats, The; Diane Stein (1994)

Nature of Animal Healing, The: The Definitive Holistic Medicine Guide to Caring for Your Dog and Cat; Martin Goldstein (2000)
Protect Your Pet: More Shocking Facts; Ann M. Martin (2001)
Veterinary Epidemiology; M. V. Thrushfield, Giuseppe Bertola, Michael Thrushfield (2005)
Welfare Of Cats, The; Irene Rochlitz (2005)

INTERNET SITES

American Animal Hospital Association
www.aahanet.org

American Veterinary Medical Association
www.avma.org

American Association of Feline Practitioners
www.aafponline.org

Colorado State University Animal Cancer Center
www.csuanimalcancercenter.org

Louisiana State University School of Veterinary Medicine/Teaching Hospitals
www.vetmed.lsu.edu/vth&c/default.htm

Cornell University Hospital For Animals
www.vet.cornell.edu/hospital/companion.htm

University of Wisconsin-Madison Veterinary Medical Teaching Hospital
http://vmthpub.vetmed.wisc.edu/sa_services

Shirley's Wellness Café
www.shirleys-wellness-cafe.com/animals.htm

Vet Info
www.vetinfo.com

The Pet Center
www.thepetcenter.com/exa/vac.html

HolistiCat
www.holisticat.com/vaccinations.html

Index

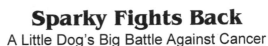

ORDER FORM

To order additional copies of this book, simply fill in this form and mail with payment.

Please send me _____ copies of
Stop The Shots! : Are Vaccinations Killing Our Pets?

How many copies?	Cost ($8.95 + $2.00 S/H **per copy**)	Total Enclosed (Check or Money Order Only)
	x $10.95	

Ship via USPS Mail.

<u>Note</u>: US and Canadian orders only. Other countries please purchase online at *www.StopTheShots.com*

PLEASE PRINT CLEARLY:

Full Name	
Address 1	
Address 2	
City	State
Zip Code	
Email	
Telephone (day): [ ] [ ]	
Area Number	

Send to:
Foley Square Books
P. O. Box 20548, Park West Station
New York, NY 10025

CPSIA information can be obtained
at www.ICGtesting.com
Printed in the USA
BVHW01s1340201217
503317BV00001B/19/P